# Shadows of Absence:

*Journeys Through Loss and Resilience*

*Rae Maker*

## *TABLE OF CONTENTS*

# Introduction

In the quiet spaces of our lives, where laughter once resided and memories were made, there often comes a silence that is both profound and deeply unsettling. This silence doesn't announce its arrival; it creeps in, filling the rooms and hearts with a presence that is both palpable and invisible. It's the silence that follows the storm, the quiet that comes after the battle has been fought—not with swords and shields, but with hope, tears, and the relentless march of time against an enemy that knows no mercy: cancer.

My name is Rae Maker, and I have lived through this silence more times than any heart should bear. I have been the one left standing, the one left to navigate the aftermath of a war that took from me not one, but three beloved companions. Two of my wives were taken by cancer, leaving behind a tapestry of memories and a world that suddenly seemed too vast and empty without them.

This book is for those of us who have loved deeply, fought bravely alongside those we cherish, and ultimately, faced the agony of their absence. It's for the husbands, wives, children, and friends who have stood in the shadow of cancer, feeling both its chill and the warmth of the love that refuses to fade. Shadows of Absence: Journeys Through Loss and Resilience is not just a recounting of loss; it's a narrative about the other victims of cancer—the ones who don't appear in medical reports or statistics but whose lives are irrevocably changed by this disease. It's about the struggle, the pain, and the profound resilience of the human spirit. Through this book, I hope to offer a hand to hold in the dark, a whisper of understanding in the silence, and perhaps, a guide to finding a path through grief. The journey of cancer is not walked alone. Besides every person who faces this formidable foe, there is a network of lives touched, changed, and sometimes shattered by the experience.

From the moment of diagnosis, life as we know it is altered. We enter a world filled with terms we wish we didn't understand, treatments that bring both hope and hardship and the ever-present shadow of uncertainty. This book will walk you through the beginning of the end, where normalcy is a distant memory, and every day is a lesson in love, strength, and endurance. But even in the darkest of times, there are moments of grace. There are instances where the human spirit shines so brightly, illuminating the depths of love and compassion we are capable of.

These moments are treasures, glimmers of light in a journey marked by shadows. They remind us that even amid pain, there is beauty, and even in the heart of loss, there is something to be gained. The role of the caregiver is often a mantle taken up with love but carried with a weight that can feel insurmountable. This book delves into the silent battles fought by those who stand by, offering their strength, their time, and often, pieces of their own health and well-being to the altar of hope. It's a testament to the unseen sacrifices and the unspoken struggles that weave through the fabric of caregiving. As the journey progresses towards its inevitable end, we are faced with the reality of saying goodbye.

This book explores the complexity of emotions that accompany the farewell, the desire to hold on and the necessity of letting go. It's a conversation about dignity, about love, and about the profound act of releasing someone we cannot imagine living without. And then, there's the aftermath—the silence after the storm. This book seeks to navigate the landscape of loss, a terrain that is as varied as it is vast.

Grief does not come with a map, nor does it adhere to a timeline. It's a journey of its own, marked by unexpected detours, moments of despair, and instances of unexpected beauty. In sharing this path, I hope to offer solace, understanding, and perhaps a way to weave the threads of loss into the fabric of our lives, making it not just stronger, but more beautiful for the scars. But loss is not the end of the story. It's a chapter that, once lived, becomes a part of us—shaping, changing, and ultimately, contributing to the narrative of our lives.

This book is also about the legacy left by those we've lost—the lessons they've taught us, the love they've given us, and how they continue to influence our journey. It's about carrying their memory forward, not just as a shadow of absence, but as a beacon of love, resilience, and hope. In the final chapters, we look beyond the personal stories to the broader picture—the community of support that exists for those touched by cancer, the advances in research that offer hope for the future, and the ways in which our pain can be transformed into purpose. It's a testament to the strength of the human spirit, the power of community, and the enduring light of hope. Shadows of Absence: Journeys Through Loss and Resilience is more than just my story or the story of my loved ones. It's a reflection of the collective journey of all who have loved someone with cancer. It's a conversation about loss, love, and the indomitable will to keep moving forward, carrying with us the memories of those we've lost, and the lessons they've taught us about living. As you turn these pages, my hope is that you find within them something that resonates—a word, a story, a moment—that offers comfort, understanding, or perhaps a new perspective on your own journey. You are not alone in the shadows. Together, we walk this path, guided by the love of those we've lost and the shared hope for a future where cancer no longer has the power to leave us in the silence of absence.

# Chapter 1:

# The Diagnosis - The Beginning of

# the End

### 1.1 Shockwaves Through Normalcy

You know, there's something about the word "normal" that we all take for granted. It's like this comfortable, predictable pattern of life that we wrap around ourselves, not realizing how fragile it is. That is, until something comes along and shatters it into a million pieces. And I'm not talking about the small stuff, like a flat tire on your way to work or a missed flight. I'm talking about the kind of thing that stops you in your tracks, that turns your world upside down. The kind of thing like a cancer diagnosis.

Imagine, just for a second, you're going about your day, the same way you always do. You're thinking about what to make for dinner, maybe planning a weekend getaway, or just trying to get through a mountain of emails. Then, suddenly, you're sitting in a doctor's office, and you hear the words that seem to echo through every corner of your existence: "It's cancer." It's like a bomb goes off in the middle of your life. Everything important a moment ago fades into the background, and now, there's just this.

The first wave that hits you is shock. It's this numb, disbelieving sensation where you're hearing the words, but they don't quite make sense. It's like your brain refuses to connect the dots because, in your world, cancer happens to other people, not to you or someone you love. Then, as the shock starts to wear off, it's replaced by this heavy, sinking feeling in your stomach. Denial kicks in, hard and fast. You start to think there's been a mistake, that maybe they mixed up the test results, or it's just a bad dream that you'll wake up from.

But as reality starts to seep in, you find yourself scrambling for information, for something, anything, that can give you a shred of hope. You dive into the internet, devouring articles, research papers, and forum posts, trying to understand this enemy that has invaded your life. Medical terms you've never heard of before become part of your daily vocabulary. Words like "metastasis," "chemotherapy," and "prognosis" are suddenly as familiar to you as the back of your hand.

And amid this chaos, this frantic search for answers, something remarkable happens. You start to see the strength of the human spirit, your spirit. You realize that even in the face of something as terrifying as cancer, you're not willing to give up. Not yet. So, you rally the troops. Family, friends, even strangers who've been through the same thing become your allies. You find comfort in their stories, their advice, and their presence. Support groups, online communities, and cancer care teams become your new normal. They're your lifeline, offering you a sense of solidarity and understanding that you can't find anywhere else.

You know, talking about cancer and its initial impact like this might make it seem all doom and gloom. But, believe it or not, there's this underlying current of hope that starts to emerge. Amidst the fear and the uncertainty, there's this determination to fight, to cling to every possible chance of beating this thing. It's not about denying the seriousness of the diagnosis, but about refusing to let it define you or your loved ones.

As we walk through this chapter together, keep in mind that it's not just a story of loss and despair. It's a story about people, about us, facing one of life's toughest battles and finding strength we never knew we had. It's about the shockwaves that disrupt our normalcy, yes, but it's also about how we learn to ride those waves, how we adapt, and how we support each other through it all. Because, at the end of the day, that's what makes us human – our ability to face the unthinkable and somehow, somehow, find a path forward.

## 1.2 The Learning Curve

You know, there's this moment after the initial shock of a cancer diagnosis, right? It's like you've been dropped into the middle of an ocean, and you're trying to figure out which way is up. This, my friend, is where the learning curve begins. And let me tell you, it's steep. You go from zero to a hundred in no time, trying to wrap your head around what's happening.

You're standing there, or maybe sitting, and the doctor starts throwing out these terms that sound like they're straight out of a sci-fi novel. Biopsy, staging, oncology – it's like learning a new language overnight. And not just any language, but one where every word could potentially change the course of your life. It's overwhelming, to say the least.

But here's the thing: humans are incredibly adaptable creatures. Faced with this mountain of information, you start to climb. You begin with the basics, understanding the type of cancer we're dealing with. Is it aggressive? What stage is it? What are the treatment options? Each question leads to a dozen more, and before you know it, you're deep in the weeds of medical research, trying to understand the pros and cons of chemotherapy versus radiation, or the potential of targeted therapy.

And it's not just the medical stuff, right? There's this whole logistical side to managing a life-threatening illness that nobody talks about. It's like suddenly, you're not just a family member or a friend; you're also a part-time medical researcher, a scheduler, a transporter, a negotiator with insurance companies. You find yourself juggling appointments, managing medications, and figuring out how to make life work around this giant curveball.

Let's not forget the emotional rollercoaster. One minute you're in research mode, feeling like you've got a handle on things, and the next, you're hit with the reality of the situation, feeling utterly lost and scared. It's a constant push and pull, trying to stay informed and make the best decisions while also dealing with the emotional weight of cancer.

But amidst this chaos, something remarkable happens. You start to find your footing. You learn to ask the right questions, to advocate for the best care, and to navigate the healthcare system like a pro. It's not easy, and it's certainly not quick, but gradually, you become more confident in your ability to manage this new reality.

And let's talk about the support networks for a second. They're like this hidden superpower that you don't realize you have until you need it. There are support groups, both in-person and online, filled with people who have been exactly where you are. They're there to offer advice, share their experiences, and just listen when you need to vent. These connections become a lifeline, offering insights and tips that you won't find in any medical textbook.

You also learn to lean on your friends and family in ways you never thought possible. They become an integral part of this journey, offering to help with the mundane tasks that suddenly become monumental, providing a shoulder to cry on, or just being there to sit in silence when that's all you can handle. It's through this network of support that you start to realize you're not alone in this.

And here's an unexpected twist: through this learning curve, you start to see the world a bit differently. Every small victory, like a successful round of treatment or a good day amidst the bad, becomes a cause for celebration. You learn to cherish the moments, to find joy in the midst of hardship, and to never take a single day for granted.

While this learning curve is steep, and at times it feels insurmountable, it's also filled with moments of incredible growth and understanding. You learn about the resilience of the human spirit, the depth of your own strength, and the incredible power of love and support.

In the end, the learning curve in the face of cancer is not just about understanding the disease; it's about understanding ourselves, our capacity for resilience, and the incredible strength we possess when faced with life's greatest challenges. It's a journey that nobody would choose, but one that teaches us more about life, love, and perseverance than we could have ever imagined.

## 1.3 Rallying the Troops

Alright, so we've navigated the shock of the diagnosis and clawed our way up the steep learning curve. Now, we find ourselves standing at the edge of something that feels a lot like going into battle. It's daunting, terrifying even, but there's this moment – this incredibly powerful moment – when you realize you're not going to face it alone. This is where we start "Rallying the Troops," and let me tell you, it's a game-changer.

Rallying the troops isn't just about sending out an SOS to every person you've ever met. It's about connecting with the people who genuinely want to stand by you through the storm. It's your family, your friends, the neighbor you only used to nod to in the morning, and even strangers who've been through the same fire and come out the other side. Suddenly, your small army begins to form, and with it, a sense of hope starts to flicker.

Now, the thing about rallying the troops is, it's not just a call to arms; it's an invitation into your heart. It's saying, "Hey, this is going to be one of the toughest things I've ever faced, and I need you." And you know what? People step up. They bring meals, offer rides to appointments, take turns sitting with you during chemotherapy sessions, or just send messages of support that become little lifelines in your darkest moments.

But it's not all logistics and practical help. Oh no. The emotional support you receive becomes this incredible force, like a shield against the onslaught of fear and uncertainty cancer brings.

There's something about knowing you're not alone in the fight that gives you a strength you never knew you had. It's the texts at just the right moment, the listening ear after a tough appointment, or the shared laughter in the midst of pain that remind you of the resilience of the human spirit.

Now, let's not sugarcoat it. Rallying the troops can also be challenging. It means being vulnerable, letting people see you at your weakest, and accepting help when every fiber of your being screams to maintain independence. But it's in this vulnerability that true connections are forged. You start to learn the incredible value of leaning on others, of being part of a community that lifts you up when you're too tired to stand on your own.

One of the most remarkable aspects of rallying the troops is how it can extend beyond your immediate circle. Support groups, whether in person or online, become a vital part of your network. Here, you find people who truly understand what you're going through because they're walking the same path. They offer advice, share their stories of hope and resilience, and become a sounding board for all the fears and frustrations that you might not want to burden your loved ones with.

And then there's the role of healthcare professionals – your medical team becomes an integral part of your troop. Building a good relationship with them, understanding that they're not just there to administer treatment but to support you through this journey, becomes key. They're the strategists in this battle, equipping you with the knowledge and tools you need to fight.

But rallying the troops is also about something deeper. It's about creating a legacy of love, support, and community. It's about showing the world, and perhaps even ourselves, what we're capable of when we come together. The troops you rally become a testament to the idea that even in our darkest hours, we are never truly alone.

Through this process, we learn not just about the generosity of others, but also about our own capacity to give, to share our vulnerabilities, and to be part of something bigger than ourselves. It teaches us that strength doesn't always come from holding on, but often from letting go and allowing others to share the load.

In essence, rallying the troops is about harnessing the power of human connection to face one of life's most formidable challenges. It's a journey that highlights the beauty of community, the strength found in vulnerability, and the indomitable spirit of those who come together to support one another. And in the midst of the battle, it's these connections, these moments of shared strength and compassion, that shine the brightest, reminding us of the incredible power of coming together in the face of adversity.

# Chapter 2

# The Battlefront - Living with Cancer

Welcome to a chapter that many of us wish we didn't have to write, yet here we are, standing on the battlefront of living with cancer. In the previous chapter, we talked about the shock of diagnosis and the incredible journey of rallying our troops. Now, it's time to delve into the daily life on this new, unchosen path. This part of the story, "Daily Struggles," is where the reality of cancer becomes a constant companion, weaving its way into the fabric of everyday life.

The daily struggles of living with cancer are as varied as they are challenging. It's not just about the big battles—the surgeries, the rounds of chemotherapy, or radiation. It's the small skirmishes that occur in the quiet moments of the day: the side effects that linger long after treatment, the fatigue that turns simple tasks into Herculean efforts, and the constant, nagging worry about what the future holds.

Let's talk about the physical toll first. Cancer and its treatment can feel like they're taking over your body. There are days when you might not recognize yourself in the mirror, when the person staring back at you is a shadow of your former self. The side effects of treatment—nausea, pain, hair loss, and so much more—become your unwelcome companions, reminding you every day of the battle you're fighting.

But it's not just a physical battle; it's an emotional one, too. There's this rollercoaster of emotions that you ride every single day. Hope and despair sit side by side, fighting for space in your heart. There are moments of fear so intense that they take your breath away, followed by moments of profound gratitude for the simple act of waking up in the morning. It's a constant tug-of-war between wanting to stay strong for your loved ones and needing to allow yourself the vulnerability to break down.

Then there's the challenge of trying to maintain some semblance of normalcy in a life that feels anything but normal. How do you go about your day-to-day life when every moment is overshadowed by cancer? You adapt. You find new ways to enjoy the things you love, even if it's in a smaller, quieter way. You celebrate the good days and brace yourself for the bad ones, knowing that both are part of this journey.

One of the hardest daily struggles, though, is dealing with uncertainty. Cancer has this way of making you question everything about your future. Plans that once seemed so certain now hang in the balance, and not knowing can be one of the toughest parts to handle. You learn to live in the moment, yes, but the shadow of uncertainty is always lurking, making even the simplest plans feel like a gamble.

But here's the thing: amidst all these struggles, there's also this incredible resilience that emerges. You start to find strength in places you never knew existed, both within yourself and in the world around you. You learn to appreciate the little victories— a good test result, a day without nausea, a moment of laughter amidst the tears. These small triumphs become beacons of hope, guiding you through the darkest days.

Living with cancer is also about redefining what it means to live fully. It's about finding joy in the simplest of moments, cherishing the time with loved ones, and appreciating the beauty in the world in a way you never did before. It's a harsh teacher, cancer, but the lessons it teaches about life, love, and resilience are invaluable.

While the daily struggles of living with cancer are real and relentless, they're also interspersed with moments of profound beauty and strength. It's a journey that tests you in ways you never imagined, but it's also one that reveals the incredible capacity of the human spirit to endure, adapt, and find light in the darkest of places.

As we move on, remember that it's not just a story of hardship and pain. It's also a story of resilience, hope, and the indomitable will to keep moving forward, one day at a time. It's a reminder that even on the battlefront of living with cancer, there can be moments of grace, beauty, and profound strength.

## 2.2 Moments of Grace

As we continue navigating the rugged terrain of living with cancer, amidst the daily struggles and relentless battles, there emerges a surprising, often unexpected phenomenon: Moments of Grace. These are the instances that light up the darkness, offering a profound sense of peace, joy, and connection. They remind us of the beauty and resilience of the human spirit. Let's look into these moments, uncovering the silver linings that cancer, despite its best efforts, cannot tarnish.

### The Power of Presence

In the thick of cancer's chaos, the simple act of being present takes on a new, profound meaning. There's a grace in the quiet companionship of a friend sitting beside you during a chemo session, not saying anything, just being there. Real-life stories abound of individuals who've felt isolated in their journey, only to find solace in the silent, steadfast presence of a loved one. Like the young mother who, weakened by treatment, was silently supported by her husband, who took over all household duties without a word, his actions a powerful testament to unconditional love and partnership.

### Unexpected Joys

Cancer sharpens the focus on life's small pleasures, transforming them into significant sources of joy. Consider the tale of a man who found immense happiness in the taste of ice cream after weeks of battling nausea and loss of appetite. Or the woman who, having lost her hair to chemotherapy, was moved to tears by the gentle touch of rain on her scalp—a sensation she'd never thought to cherish. These moments, small as they may seem, act as potent reminders of the beauty that persists in our world, even in times of great pain.

## Strength in Vulnerability

There's an unexpected grace in vulnerability, in the willingness to open up about fears, hopes, and the reality of living with cancer. This openness can forge deeper connections with others, creating a space for genuine support and understanding. A poignant example is found in support groups, where strangers, bound by their shared struggles, become lifelines for each other, offering empathy, encouragement, and a listening ear. Stories of these connections often highlight how sharing one's vulnerability can lead to powerful, life-affirming relationships.

## Redefining Success

The journey with cancer brings a shift in perspective on what constitutes success. Suddenly, the small victories—a successful round of treatment, a good day amidst the bad—become monumental achievements. There's grace in celebrating these moments, in recognizing the immense courage and resilience they represent. A father who, after a grueling treatment session, musters the energy to attend his daughter's school play, finds joy and triumph not in grand achievements but in being present for those he loves.

## Legacy of Love

Perhaps the most profound moments of grace emerge in the reflection on the legacy left by those who face cancer. It's in the stories they share, the lessons they impart, and the love they spread. Like the young woman who, in the final stages of her battle, dedicated her time to writing letters to her loved ones, expressing her love, hopes, and dreams for them. Her legacy, a testament to the enduring power of love, continues to inspire and comfort her family, transforming grief into a celebration of her life.

## A New Dawn

Cancer, for all its darkness, can lead to a renewed appreciation for life. Survivors often speak of a "new normal" that includes a deeper gratitude for each new day, a heightened awareness of life's fragility, and a commitment to living more fully and purposefully. This renewed outlook can be a powerful force for good, inspiring others to cherish their lives and the people in them more deeply.

## Embracing the Moments

Moments of grace amidst the cancer journey are like beacons of light, guiding us through the storm. They remind us that, even in the face of immense challenge, there is beauty, love, and strength to be found. By embracing these moments, we acknowledge the complexity of the human experience—marked by pain, yes, but also by incredible resilience and an indomitable will to find joy and meaning in every circumstance.

## 2.3 The Caregiver's Burden

Let's talk about a group of heroes who often fly under the radar in the whole cancer saga—the caregivers. You know, the spouses, family members, and friends who step into the breach, day in, day out, without a second thought. This part of the journey, "The Caregiver's Burden," is their story. It's about the weight they carry, a load that's as heavy as it is invisible to the outside world.

### The Invisible Load

First off, being a caregiver isn't something most sign up for; it's a role thrust upon them by circumstance. And it's a marathon, not a sprint. Imagine juggling your job, and family life, and then adding the full-time job of caring for someone with cancer. It's like being asked to keep multiple plates spinning, knowing if one drops, it could shatter everything. Caregivers often put their lives on pause, bearing a silent, relentless strain that's hard to articulate.

### The Emotional Rollercoaster

Let's not sugarcoat it—the emotional toll on caregivers is profound. They ride the same rollercoaster of hope and despair as the person they're caring for, but often, they feel they must hide their fears to stay strong for their loved ones. There's guilt, too, lurking in the shadows. Guilt for feeling overwhelmed, for yearning for a semblance of their old life, and even guilt for being healthy. It's a constant battle between their heart and mind, trying to navigate their own emotions while being a rock for someone else.

## Physical Toll and Social Isolation

Physically, the demands can be just as taxing. Sleepless nights, long hospital stays, the physical act of caring for someone—it all adds up, wearing down the caregiver's health. Then there's the social isolation. Friends who don't know what to say start to drift away; social activities become a thing of the past. The world seems to shrink to the size of the cancer battle, leaving caregivers feeling cut off from the life they once knew.

## Finding Support

But here's where the plot twists. In the midst of all this, caregivers find strength they never knew they had. They learn to lean on support groups, finding solace in sharing their experiences with those who truly understand. There's this unspoken bond that forms, a recognition that they're not alone in this fight. And sometimes, just knowing that can be enough to light the way through the darkest days.

## The Power of Small Victories

Caregivers also become masters of celebrating small victories. A good day for their loved one, a smile, a moment of relief from pain—these become monumental. They learn to live in the moment, cherishing the good times, however fleeting. It's about finding joy in the journey, no matter how rocky the road.

## The Lesson in Resilience

What's remarkable about caregivers is their resilience. Sure, they have moments of doubt, times when they feel they can't go on. But they do. They keep showing up, day after day, because their love and commitment run deep. It's a testament to the human spirit, this ability to keep going even when the going gets tough.

## A Two-Way Street

And let's not forget, the care they give often goes both ways. The person they're caring for offers them strength, too, in ways that are hard to quantify. It's in the shared laughter, the silent understanding, and the mutual appreciation for the bond that cancer, for all its cruelty, has deepened. It's a reminder that, in the heart of struggle, there's a beauty and connection that endure.

## Carving Out Self-Care

One of the toughest lessons for caregivers is learning the importance of self-care. It feels counterintuitive, like they're taking something away from their loved one. But here's the truth: taking care of themselves is what allows them to keep caring for someone else. It's not selfish; it's necessary. Whether it's a walk outside, a coffee with a friend, or just a few moments of quiet, these small acts of self-care become lifelines, helping them replenish their reserves of strength and resilience.

## The Unseen Heroes

To all the caregivers out there, navigating the complex terrain of cancer alongside their loved ones, know this: your strength is awe-inspiring. Your journey is one of unsung heroism, marked by love, sacrifice, and incredible resilience. The burden you carry may often feel invisible to the world, but it's recognized, it's valued, and above all, it's deeply appreciated. You're not just caregivers; you're warriors in your own right, fighting a battle that demands every ounce of your courage and heart. And for that, you have the utmost respect and gratitude.

# Chapter 3

# The Long Goodbye - Approaching the End

We've navigated the initial shockwaves, the steep learning curves, and those day-to-day battles that come with living with cancer. Together, we've stood shoulder to shoulder on the frontlines, marveling at those unexpected moments of grace and acknowledging the heavy load carried by the incredible caregivers. Now, we're stepping into a chapter that, honestly, I wish we could skip. But it's an essential part of the journey—Chapter 3: "The Long Goodbye - Approaching the End."

This is the chapter that no one wants to write and even fewer want to read. It's about that phase when the treatments, the trials, and the hope of a turnaround start to wane, and the reality begins to settle in. The battle with cancer, as fierce and as fought with love and determination as it was, is drawing to a close.

Let's take a deep breath here. This part of the journey is tough, incredibly tough. It's where the physical and emotional landscapes shift dramatically. The focus moves from fighting the disease to ensuring comfort, from chasing a cure to cherishing every moment left. It's a profound, often heartbreaking transition, but also one that's filled with deep love, reflection, and, in its own way, a kind of peace.

The Long Goodbye is about preparing to part ways with someone you can't imagine your life without. It's about those conversations you never thought you'd have—conversations filled with love, sometimes regret, and often, heartfelt reflections on the journey you've shared. It's about saying those things left unsaid, about mending bridges, and creating a space where it's okay to let go, even when every fiber of your being wants to hold on tighter.

But let me tell you, amidst the sadness, there's also something incredibly beautiful about this chapter. It's in the way families come together, setting aside differences, united in their love and support. It's in the way friends rally, bringing laughter and comfort into days that seem too heavy to bear. It's in the quiet moments, the simple acts of holding a hand, sharing a favorite song, or recounting cherished memories.

Approaching the end is also about honoring the wishes of the one you love. It's about palliative care, making decisions that focus on comfort and quality of life. It's a time when the medical conversations shift, and the emphasis is on ensuring dignity and minimizing pain. And let's not forget the role of hospice care, a resource of immeasurable value, offering support and guidance through this final leg of the journey.

This chapter is a testament to the strength of the human spirit, to the power of love to shine through even in the darkest of times. It's about learning to navigate grief, to understand that it doesn't follow a neat pattern or timeline. Grief is as individual as the person experiencing it, a path that we each walk in our own way.

The Long Goodbye is a chapter of preparation, not just for the inevitable loss but for the aftermath. It's about beginning to understand that life will go on, albeit in a form that's forever altered by the absence of someone dearly loved. It's about laying the groundwork for healing, for remembering, and eventually, finding a way to move forward.

As we step into this chapter, remember, that you're not alone. The emotions, the struggles, and the moments of peace you'll encounter here are shared by many who've walked this path before you. Together, we'll explore the complexities of approaching the end with grace, love, and resilience. And together, we'll learn how to say goodbye in a way that honors the life, the love, and the legacy of those we're preparing to let go.

## 3.1 Facing Mortality

Here we are, at a place on this journey that's both deeply personal and universally inevitable—facing mortality. It's a chapter we all read with a heavy heart, knowing that it's about coming to terms with the end of a life story. It's about facing the reality that, despite all our advances in medicine, technology, and knowledge, we're all mortal.

When cancer enters the picture, this realization often comes much sooner than we'd ever expect or want. It's like being on a road you thought you knew well, only to find it abruptly ends, leaving you standing at the edge of an unknown precipice. It's a stark, sometimes terrifying place to be, not just for the person with cancer, but for everyone who loves them.

### Real-life stories of facing mortality

Take, for instance, the story of Sarah and Tom. Tom was diagnosed with an aggressive form of cancer that left them both reeling. They had plans, and dreams of growing old together, traveling the world, and watching their grandchildren grow up. Suddenly, those dreams were overshadowed by a timeline they couldn't control. Facing Tom's mortality meant not just dealing with the practicalities of care and treatment but also grappling with the emotional weight of an impending goodbye.

Then there's the story of Mr. Chen, a gentle soul who, after a long battle with cancer, chose to spend his remaining days at home, surrounded by family. His journey of facing mortality was one of quiet acceptance. He found solace in small moments— watching the sunrise, enjoying the company of his loved ones, sharing stories of his youth. For Mr. Chen, facing mortality was about finding peace in the life he had lived and the legacy he would leave behind.

## The emotional landscape

The process of facing mortality is fraught with emotions. There's fear, of course—the fear of the unknown, of leaving loved ones behind, of pain and suffering. But there's also room for love, deeper and more poignant than ever. Conversations turn more heartfelt, with words of love, forgiveness, and sometimes, reconciliation being shared in the quiet moments.

Anger can surface, too, a natural response to a life being cut short. It's okay to feel angry, to question the fairness of it all. And amidst these swirling emotions, moments of profound joy and laughter can still find their way in, reminding us that even in the shadow of mortality, life continues to offer its gifts.

## The gift of time

One thing that becomes crystal clear is the value of time. Every moment becomes precious, not in a clichéd way, but genuinely, deeply precious. People facing their mortality often speak of a heightened awareness of the present, of a desire to live fully in the time they have left. It's a lesson for us all, really, about the fragility of life and the importance of cherishing each day.

## Preparing and saying goodbye

Facing mortality also involves the tough but necessary conversations about end-of-life wishes. It's about making sure that the person's desires for their final days are known and respected. These conversations, though incredibly hard, can also be filled with love and respect, offering a sense of control in a situation that feels anything but.

And then, there's saying goodbye. It's not just about the final words or gestures, but about all the ways we show our love and appreciation for someone's presence in our lives. It's a process, one that doesn't end with a final breath but continues in the hearts and memories of those who remain.

## Carrying forward

In facing mortality, there's also a forward-looking aspect. It's about how we carry the essence of the person with us, how their life influences ours even after they're gone. It's about finding ways to honor their memory, to continue their legacy in big and small ways.

Facing mortality is, undoubtedly, one of the hardest chapters in the cancer journey. It's a testament to the strength and resilience of the human spirit, a reminder of the depth of our capacity for love and compassion. It teaches us about the beauty of life, the importance of forgiveness, and the unbreakable bonds of family and friendship. And while it's a chapter we all wish we could skip, it's also one that brings invaluable lessons about what it truly means to live.

## 3.2 Palliative Care and Comfort

Welcome to a part of the journey that's all about compassion, care, and comfort—Palliative Care and Comfort. After facing the stark reality of mortality, we find ourselves in a space where the focus shifts from battling the disease to ensuring the highest quality of life for whatever time remains. It's a gentle, yet profoundly significant transition that centers on providing relief from the symptoms and stress of a serious illness. Let's dive into what this means, shall we?

### Understanding Palliative Care

Palliative care is a beautiful concept that sometimes gets misunderstood. It's not about giving up; it's about choosing to live as well as possible for as long as possible. It's a multidisciplinary approach that addresses not just the physical pain, but also the emotional, spiritual, and social needs of both the patient and their family. Imagine a team of doctors, nurses, therapists, and social workers, all coming together with the sole purpose of making the journey as comfortable and fulfilling as it can be.

Take, for example, Maria, who was diagnosed with advanced cancer. The introduction of palliative care into her treatment plan didn't mean her team stopped treating her cancer. Instead, it meant they started treating her as a whole person. They managed her pain, helped her with fatigue, and addressed her anxiety, allowing her moments of peace and the ability to enjoy time with her loved ones.

## The Role of Comfort Care

Comfort care is a crucial part of palliative care, focusing on relieving symptoms and improving quality of life. It's about creating an environment where the person feels supported, understood, and, most importantly, comfortable. This could mean managing pain with medication, providing physical therapy to ease discomfort, or offering nutritional support to combat weakness.

But it's also about the less tangible forms of comfort. It's the music therapy sessions that bring a smile to someone's face, the pet visits that light up a room, or the spiritual counseling that offers solace. It's about recognizing and honoring the person's life, their joys, and their fears, ensuring they feel valued and loved.

## Decisions and Conversations

A significant part of palliative care involves having those tough conversations about end-of-life wishes and making decisions that align with the individual's values and preferences. This is about empowerment—giving the person a voice in their care, even when they might feel most vulnerable.

John, for instance, chose to focus his remaining time on quality rather than quantity. With the support of his palliative care team, he made informed decisions about which treatments he wanted to continue and which he preferred to stop. These decisions allowed him to spend his final weeks at home, surrounded by family, in a familiar and comforting environment.

## The Importance of Family and Caregiver Support

Palliative care extends its compassionate embrace to the family and caregivers, recognizing the immense emotional toll the journey takes on them. It offers respite care, counseling, and support groups, providing a much-needed space for them to express their feelings, find support, and learn how to navigate their own grief and stress.

## Finding Peace in Palliative Care

Perhaps the most profound aspect of palliative care is its ability to bring peace to a tumultuous time. It's about acknowledging the inevitable while striving to make every day as good as it can be. It's finding those moments of joy, laughter, and love amidst the pain and uncertainty.

For Emma, whose father received palliative care in his final months, it was the peace of knowing he was comfortable, free from pain, and able to share precious moments with his family that meant the world. It was the gentle nights of storytelling, the shared meals, and the quiet understanding that, though the journey was ending, it was ending on their terms.

## A Testament to Human Dignity

Palliative care and comfort care stand as a testament to the dignity of every human life. They remind us that, even in the face of death, there can be beauty, grace, and peace. They teach us that caring for someone in their most vulnerable moments is one of the highest forms of love and humanity.

As we navigate this gentle chapter, let's remember the value of palliative care in honoring the person's journey, providing comfort, and upholding dignity until the very end. It's a reminder that, in the darkest of times, there is light to be found in the care, compassion, and comfort we provide to one another.

## 3.3 The Final Days

Heading into "The Final Days" is like walking through a quiet, sacred space in the forest of life's journey. It's here, in these tender, bittersweet moments, that the world seems to slow down a bit, allowing space for reflection, love, and an indescribable depth of connection. It's a chapter that many of us approach with a heavy heart, knowing it signifies the close of a precious life story. Yet, within this solemn time, there's an unexpected beauty and peace to be found. Let's talk about what this time can mean for those we love and for ourselves.

### Embracing Each Moment

In the final days, time takes on a new meaning. It's no longer about the future or the past but about the deep, rich presence of now. Every moment shared every touch, every look, becomes a treasure. There's a story I heard about Ellen and her grandmother in her final days. They spent hours just sitting together, holding hands, sometimes talking, sometimes just being in silence. Ellen said those quiet hours felt like a lifetime of love condensed into each minute. It's in these final days that we truly learn the value of presence, of simply being there for one another, without distractions, fully engaged and heart open.

## Navigating the Waves of Emotion

The emotional landscape during this time is complex and varied. There's sadness, of course, a profound grief for the impending loss. But there can also be moments of profound gratitude for the life shared, for the love given and received. It's okay to feel a wide range of emotions, from relief that their suffering will end, to anger that they're leaving, to peace in moments of quiet connection. It's all part of the human experience, this tapestry of feelings that makes up our relationships.

## Creating a Comfortable Environment

The focus on comfort and peace extends beyond the emotional to the physical environment. It's about making the space as calming and soothing as possible. Soft lighting, gentle music, familiar scents—all these can create a sanctuary that soothes the soul and eases the transition. I remember a family who turned their living room into a cozy haven filled with photos, favorite books, and even recordings of birdsong, transforming it into a place of peace and memory for their loved one's final days.

## The Role of Palliative Care

Palliative care becomes a guiding light in these final days, ensuring that pain is managed, that dignity is maintained, and that the family feels supported. The care team becomes an extension of the family, offering not just medical care but emotional and spiritual support as well. It's a partnership, one that honors the person's life and eases the journey for everyone involved.

## Saying Goodbye

Perhaps the most challenging part of the final days is saying goodbye. It's not just a single moment but a series of small releases, of letting go, of expressing love in its most pure and simple form. It's about finding the words or gestures that convey what's in your heart, even when your heart is breaking.

A beautiful example comes from a young man, Alex, who spent the last days with his partner writing letters to each other, sharing memories, hopes, and affirmations of love. For them, this act of writing was a way to say goodbye, a tangible expression of their bond that would last beyond death.

## The Gift of the Final Days

As paradoxical as it might sound, the final days can bring gifts. They remind us of what's truly important—love, connection, and the grace of shared humanity. They teach us about strength, about the capacity of the human heart to hold both joy and sorrow, and about the beauty of being fully present for each other.

Navigating the final days is a profoundly personal and shared journey. It's a time marked by tenderness, by a deepening of relationships, and by the acknowledgment of life's fleeting nature. And as we move through this chapter, we carry forward the love, the lessons, and the memories, allowing them to shape us, guide us, and remind us of the preciousness of every moment we have together.

# Chapter 4

# The Aftermath - Living with Loss

Alright, take a deep breath with me. We've journeyed through the diagnosis, the daily struggles, the care, and the final goodbyes. Now, we find ourselves stepping into a chapter that's as inevitable as it is painful—The Aftermath: Living with Loss. It's here, in the quiet wake of the storm, where we begin to grasp the reality of a world reshaped by absence.

The aftermath of losing someone to cancer is a landscape marked by silence—a silence that's profound, sometimes comforting, often deafening. It's like coming home to a house where every room echoes with memories, where every object, every photo, tells a story of a life deeply intertwined with yours. And suddenly, you're tasked with the unimaginable: to continue living in a world that no longer includes one of its main characters.

Living with loss is like navigating an unfamiliar terrain without a map. There are no right paths, no wrong turns, just a journey through grief that's as unique as the person you've lost. It's about learning to walk through life with a hole in your heart, finding ways to fill it not with a replacement, but with love, memories, and the lessons they've left behind.

Think of it as a new chapter in your relationship with the person you've lost. Yes, they're no longer here in the physical sense, but their influence, their love, and the ways they've shaped you continue to play a significant role in your life. It's about holding them close, not just in moments of sadness, but in moments of joy, in decisions, in milestones, acknowledging that their absence doesn't diminish their impact on your life.

In the immediate aftermath, the world expects you to go through the stages of grief as if they're neatly laid out steps to be climbed and conquered. But grief doesn't work like that. It's more like waves—sometimes you're standing strong, and other times you're knocked off your feet by a sudden memory or a date on the calendar. And that's okay. Grief doesn't adhere to a timeline. It's something you carry with you, something that evolves and changes as you do.

Amidst the loss, there's also this unexpected sense of community that emerges. You find yourself connecting with others who've walked similar paths, who understand the language of loss without needing it to be spoken. There's comfort in these connections, a reminder that you're not alone in your grief, that love and loss are universal experiences that bind us together.

Living with loss also opens up a space for reflection—on life, on love, and on the legacy of the person you've lost. It's a time when you start to see the world through a lens shaped by their influence. Maybe you find yourself adopting their optimism, their kindness, or their passion for a cause. In a way, it's a continuation of their story through you, a testament to the fact that even in death, they continue to inspire, guide, and touch lives.

As we navigate this chapter together, remember that living with loss is not about moving on or forgetting. It's about moving forward, carrying with you the love, the memories, and the lessons of the person you've lost. It's about finding ways to honor their life, to celebrate their impact, and to keep their spirit alive in your actions, your choices, and your way of being in the world.

Therefore, take it one step at a time, one breath at a time. Allow yourself to feel, to grieve, and to heal in your way, in your own time. And know that in the aftermath of loss, there's still life to be lived—a life that's richer, deeper, and more meaningful because of the love you shared.

## 4.1 The Silence After the Storm

Stepping into "The Silence After the Storm" feels like walking into a room where the music has suddenly stopped, leaving behind a quiet so profound it reverberates through every corner of your being. For me, this silence was not encountered once, but three heart-wrenching times, with the loss of my two wives to cancer. Each time, the storm of cancer raged, tore through our lives with merciless ferocity, and then, just as suddenly, left a silence in its wake—a silence filled with memories, love, and an aching absence.

## A Tapestry of Memories

Each of my wives, a unique and beautiful soul, left behind a tapestry woven with threads of joy, laughter, and love. The silence that followed their passing wasn't just the absence of their physical presence; it was the quiet of a life no longer filled with their laughter, their voice, their unique essence. It's in this silence where I found myself sitting, sometimes lost, often reflective, sifting through the memories we created together.

Remembering each of them, their courage, their strength, and the distinct way each loved and lived became a ritual in the silence. My first wife, with her unwavering optimism, taught me the power of looking for light even in the darkest times. My second, with her pragmatic approach to life, showed me the importance of living in the moment, cherishing the now without fear of what tomorrow might bring. And my third who died of a blood clot, her gentle spirit, reminded me that strength isn't always loud; sometimes, it's the quiet resolve to keep going, day after day.

## Navigating the Silence

Navigating the silence after the storm meant learning to live in a world profoundly changed by loss. It was about finding ways to keep their memory alive, not just in the quiet moments of reflection but in their everyday actions and decisions. It involved creating a new normal where their absence was a constant presence, a shadow companion in my journey forward.

In the silence, I learned the importance of community and connection. Sharing stories of my wives with friends, family, and sometimes even strangers, became a bridge over the chasms of grief. It was in these connections, these shared moments of remembrance and love, that the silence began to feel less empty, less daunting.

## The Lessons in the Silence

The silence after the storm brought with it lessons, some hard-won, others gently revealed. I learned that grief doesn't have a timeline, that it ebbs and flows like the tide, unpredictable yet constant. I discovered that healing doesn't mean forgetting but finding a way to integrate the loss into the fabric of my being, allowing it to shape me without defining me.

I also learned about resilience—the incredible human capacity to face the deepest of losses and still find a way to keep going. This resilience wasn't just about strength; it was about vulnerability, about allowing myself to feel the full weight of my grief, to acknowledge it, and to let it teach me about love, loss, and the fragile beauty of life.

## Carrying Their Legacy Forward

In the silence, I found purpose in carrying forward the legacy of my wives. Each left behind not just memories but lessons, ideals, and passions that I chose to embrace and champion. Whether it was volunteering for cancer research in honor of their battles, advocating for better patient care, or simply living life with more kindness, empathy, and joy, their legacy became a guiding light in my journey through the silence.

## Finding Peace

Finding peace in the silence after the storm is an ongoing journey, one that doesn't have a clear destination. It's about learning to live with the absence, to embrace the memories, and to find joy and meaning in a world forever changed. It's about recognizing that the love we shared doesn't end with death but continues, a constant force that guides, inspires, and comforts.

The silence after the storm, while initially a place of profound grief and loss, gradually transformed into a space of reflection, growth, and quiet strength. It became a testament to the enduring power of love—a love that, even in absence, continues to shape, define, and enrich my life in ways I'm still discovering. And so, in the silence, I carry on, guided by the memories, the lessons, and the love of three incredible women who forever changed the course of my life.

## 4.2 Navigating Grief

Navigating grief is like finding yourself in the middle of a vast, uncharted ocean. You're in a small boat, no land in sight, waves of emotions crashing against you from all directions. You've got no compass, no map, just the stars above and your own resilience to guide you. It's a journey that's both deeply personal and universally understood, a path that millions have walked, yet one that feels profoundly solitary.

### Grief's Unpredictable Waves

First off, let's get one thing straight: grief doesn't follow a neat, linear path. You might have heard about the stages of grief—denial, anger, bargaining, depression, and acceptance. But in reality, grief is more like a tangled mess of yarn than a straight line. You might feel anger one moment, acceptance the next, then back to denial. It's all normal. It's all part of the process.

Someone described her grief as a "rollercoaster in the fog." Some days, she felt almost normal, laughing at a joke or enjoying a meal. Then, suddenly, a wave of grief would hit her out of nowhere, leaving her breathless with sadness. Over time, she learned that grief wasn't something to be conquered or resolved, but something to be navigated, day by day, moment by moment.

## The Solitude of Grief

One of the toughest parts of grieving is the loneliness that often accompanies it. Even when surrounded by supportive friends and family, there's a solitude to grief that's hard to explain. It's as if you're in a room full of people, yet speaking a language only you understand.

This solitude isn't necessarily a bad thing. It can provide the space and silence needed to reflect, to mourn, and to gradually find your way through the pain. But it's also important to reach out, to share your grief with others who can offer a listening ear, a shoulder to cry on, or even just their presence.

## Finding Expression

Grief needs to be expressed, to find a way out of the heart and into the world. For some, this means talking—sharing stories of the person lost, speaking about the pain, the memories, the love. For others, expression comes through writing, painting, music, or any form of creative outlet that allows the emotions to flow.

There is the story of Alex, who took up painting after his partner died. He'd never painted before and didn't even consider himself artistic. But he found that on the canvas, he could express what he couldn't put into words. Each stroke, each color, became a testament to his love and his loss.

## Support and Solidarity

Finding support is crucial in navigating grief. Support groups, whether in person or online, can be invaluable. They offer a space where the language of loss is understood, where the waves of grief are acknowledged and shared.

But support can also come from unexpected places—from a neighbor who's experienced loss, from a colleague who reaches out, from a book that speaks to your soul. It's about finding those moments of connection that remind you, even in the deepest solitude of grief, that you're not alone.

## Growth and Transformation

Here's the thing about grief: as much as it's about loss, it's also about growth. It forces us to confront the most profound questions about life, love, and our own mortality. It challenges us, and breaks us down, but also offers the opportunity to rebuild, to find new meanings, new purposes, and new strengths.

Grief can transform us, shaping us into more compassionate, empathetic, and resilient beings. It teaches us to cherish the present, to love more deeply, and to live more fully. It's a harsh teacher, no doubt, but the lessons it imparts are some of the most valuable we'll ever learn.

## Navigating Together

Navigating grief is a journey that each of us must walk in our way, but it's also a path we don't have to walk alone. By sharing our stories, our pain, and our love, we can find solace in each other's experiences, and strength in our shared humanity.

After we chart our course through the uncharted waters of grief, let's remember to look up at the stars, to reach out to those around us, and to keep rowing, even when the shore is nowhere in sight. For in the vast ocean of grief, we find not only the depths of sorrow but also the possibility of growth, connection, and, eventually, a renewed sense of hope and purpose.

## 4.3 Rebuilding and Finding Meaning:

Now, let's dive into something a bit uplifting, shall we? We've talked about the storm, the silence that follows, and the tumultuous waves of grief. Now, we're at a chapter that's all about picking up the pieces, about finding solid ground again— Rebuilding and Finding Meaning. This is where the journey takes a turn, where the fog starts to lift, and you begin to see glimpses of a path forward.

## The Art of Rebuilding

Rebuilding after loss is like piecing together a mosaic from shattered glass. At first glance, all you see are fragments, sharp edges, and a semblance of what used to be. But as you start to pick up the pieces, you realize that you're creating something new, something unique and beautiful in its own right.

It doesn't happen overnight, and it's not without its challenges. There are days when it feels like you're making progress, like you're starting to see a picture form. Then, there are days when it all seems pointless, when the pieces don't seem to fit anywhere. That's okay. Rebuilding is not about restoring what was lost but about creating something new from the love, memories, and lessons that remain.

## Finding Meaning

One of the most profound aspects of this journey is the quest for meaning. It's about asking the big questions: Why did this happen? What's the purpose of all this pain? How do I move forward from here? The answers aren't always clear, and they often take time to surface. But in the searching, in the questioning, there's growth, there's understanding, and eventually, there's a sense of purpose that emerges.

For some, finding meaning might involve honoring the person they've lost by living out their values, continuing their work, or embracing a cause they were passionate about. I met a woman, Lisa, who started a charity in her husband's name, dedicated to the cause he cared about deeply. Through her work, she found a way to keep his spirit alive, to transform her grief into action, into something that brought hope and help to others.

## The Role of Community

As you rebuild and search for meaning, the community around you plays a pivotal role. It's in the shared stories, the mutual support, and the collective wisdom where you find strength and inspiration. Whether it's a support group, a network of friends and family, or a community of people who've faced similar losses, these connections are invaluable. They remind you that you're not alone in your journey, that others have walked this path before you, and that together, you can find a way through.

## Embracing Change

Rebuilding and finding meaning also means embracing change. It's about allowing yourself to grow, to change direction, and to be open to new possibilities. It might mean discovering new interests, pursuing new goals, or even changing the way you live your life. It's about saying yes to life, even when part of you is still holding on to what was lost.

There is a story of a father who lost his daughter to cancer. In the years that followed, he found solace in nature, something they both loved. He started hiking, something he'd never done before, and with every step, he felt closer to her, more at peace. It was a change that brought him unexpected joy and a renewed sense of connection to the world around him.

## A New Chapter

Ultimately, rebuilding and finding meaning is about writing a new chapter in your life. It's not about forgetting the past or replacing what was lost but about building upon it, creating a life that's rich, meaningful, and full of possibilities. It's about carrying the love and memories with you, letting them guide you, inspire you, and push you to live more fully, more deeply.

So, as we embark on this journey of rebuilding, let's remember that it's not just about moving on but about moving forward, with love as our compass and the memories as our guide. It's about finding light in the darkness, hope in the despair, and meaning in the loss. And in doing so, we honor those we've lost, not just in our memories, but in the way we choose to live our lives from here on out.

# Chapter 5

# The Legacy - Carrying Their Memory Forward

We've been through quite the journey together, haven't we? From the tumultuous onset of grief, navigating its unpredictable waves, to the delicate process of rebuilding and finding new meanings in life. Now, we step into a deeply resonant chapter, one that's about honoring, cherishing, and carrying forward the memories and legacies of those we've loved and lost—Chapter 5: The Legacy - Carrying Their Memory Forward.

This chapter is a celebration, a testament to the enduring impact of love and the profound ways in which our loved ones continue to influence us, even in their absence. It's about recognizing that while they may no longer be with us in physical form, their spirit, their teachings, and their essence are interwoven into the fabric of our lives, guiding us, inspiring us, and sometimes challenging us to be better, to do more, to live fully.

## The Essence of Legacy

Legacy isn't just about what's left behind; it's about what's carried forward. It's the stories we tell, the traditions we uphold, and the lessons we pass on. It's in the way we live our lives, influenced by the love we've shared and the challenges we've faced together. It's a rich, multifaceted tapestry made of memories, values, and the subtle ways our loved ones have shaped us.

After my journey through loss, I've come to see that carrying forward a legacy isn't a passive act—it's a choice, a deliberate and loving effort to keep their spirit alive. Whether it's through adopting their passion for a cause, continuing a hobby they loved, or simply embodying the qualities they exuded—kindness, resilience, joy—we ensure that their impact on the world doesn't end with their passing.

## Building Bridges

Carrying their memory forward is also about building bridges—between past and present, between grief and joy, between loss and discovery. It's about finding ways to weave their memory into the everyday, allowing their presence to be felt in the small, seemingly mundane moments, as well as the significant milestones.

I've met people who've dedicated themselves to causes their loved ones were passionate about, turning their pain into purpose. Others find solace in creative expression, painting, writing, or composing music that captures the essence of the memories they cherish. Some simply find ways to speak their loved one's name, to share stories and lessons learned, keeping their memory vibrant and alive.

## A Living Legacy

What's beautiful about carrying forward a legacy is that it evolves. It's not a static relic of the past but a living, breathing presence that grows and changes as we do. It's in the way we navigate our lives, influenced by their wisdom and buoyed by their love. It's a guiding light, helping us find our way through the darkness, encouraging us to seek joy, to embrace life, and to love deeply.

In my own journey, I've found that carrying forward the legacy of those I've lost has brought a sense of purpose, a deeper connection to the values that we shared, and a comforting sense of continuity. It's a way of honoring their life, not just through remembrance, but through action, through living a life that reflects their influence, their dreams, and their love.

## Welcoming You to This Chapter

As we embark on this chapter together, I invite you to think about the legacies of those you've lost. Consider how they've touched your life, the lessons they've imparted, and the love they've shared. Think about how you can carry their memory forward, not just as a tribute to them, but as a gift to yourself and the world.

Carrying forward a legacy is a journey of love, a way of weaving the essence of those we've lost into the ongoing story of our lives. It's a chapter that's about looking back with gratitude, living in the present with purpose, and moving forward with hope, all the while holding their memory close to our hearts. Let's explore together how we can honor and celebrate the lasting impact of those we've loved, ensuring that their legacy shines brightly, guiding us and future generations.

## 5.1 Keeping the Memory Alive

Moving through the quiet aftermath of loss and the gentle process of rebuilding, we've arrived at a deeply meaningful practice—Keeping the Memory Alive. It's in this sacred space that we find innovative and heartfelt ways to ensure that the essence of our loved ones continues to resonate, not just within us but around us, shaping our world in subtle yet profound ways.

### The Rituals of Remembrance

Creating rituals is one of the most powerful ways to keep a memory alive. These don't have to be grand gestures; often, it's the small, personal rituals that carry the most meaning. For instance, I met a woman who, every year on her late husband's birthday, would hike to their favorite spot in the local hills, a place where they shared countless sunsets and conversations. There, she'd read aloud a letter she wrote to him, catching him up on the year's events, her thoughts, her fears, and her triumphs. This ritual became a bridge between her current life and the life they shared, a moment of connection across the divide of death.

### Spaces of Memory

Creating a physical space that honors your loved one can be a tangible way to keep their memory alive. This might be a dedicated shelf in your home with photos, keepsakes, and items that were significant to them. Or perhaps a garden planted in their honor, filled with their favorite flowers or trees. Every time you tend to the plants, or simply sit and reflect in this space, you're nurturing their memory, allowing it to grow and flourish.

There is a certain family that transformed a corner of their living room into a 'memory corner' for their daughter, who loved art. They framed her paintings, displayed her sculptures, and even included art supplies for visitors to create something in her memory. This space became a source of comfort, inspiration, and connection for all who knew her.

## Telling Their Stories

Storytelling is perhaps one of the most ancient and powerful ways to keep a memory alive. Sharing stories about your loved one, whether through spoken word, writing, or digital media, allows others to see the depth of their character, the beauty of their life, and the impact they've had on those around them.

Consider writing a blog, starting a podcast, or simply sharing stories at family gatherings. Each story shared is a thread woven into the tapestry of their legacy, ensuring that their influence continues to touch lives and inspire hearts.

## Acts of Service

Channeling your grief into acts of service can transform the pain of loss into a powerful force for good. Engaging in charity work, volunteering, or starting a foundation in their name are ways to extend their influence into the world. It's about taking the love you shared and multiplying it, spreading it to others who can benefit from that warmth and kindness.

There is the story of someone who after losing a close friend to illness, a group of them came together to volunteer at a local hospice in her name. It was a way to honor her compassionate spirit and to keep her memory alive through acts of kindness and service.

## Passing Down Traditions

Traditions have a way of connecting generations, of weaving a continuous thread through the fabric of families. Keeping alive the traditions your loved one cherished is a way to honor their memory and share their legacy with future generations. It could be as simple as making their favorite recipe on special occasions, continuing a holiday tradition they started, or passing down a beloved hobby or craft.

## Digital Memorials

In our connected age, digital memorials offer a unique way to keep memories alive. Creating a website, a social media page or a digital scrapbook dedicated to your loved one allows friends and family, near and far, to contribute memories, photos, and messages. It becomes a living, evolving memorial that can reach across distances and time zones, bringing people together in remembrance and celebration.

## The Living Legacy

Keeping the memory alive is about more than just preserving the past; it's about how the essence of our loved ones inspires us to live our lives today. It's in the choices we make, the causes we support, the love we share, and the way we reach out to others in kindness and compassion. Their memory becomes a guiding light, a source of strength and inspiration, reminding us of the beauty of life, the importance of connection, and the essence of life itself.

As we explore ways to keep the memory alive, let's remember that each act of remembrance, each story shared, and each tradition upheld, is a testament to the undying impact of the ones we've lost. It's a way to ensure that their light continues to shine, illuminating our paths and warming our hearts, now and for generations to come.

## 5.2 Lessons Learned

Let's talk about something really profound that comes from our journey through loss—the lessons we learn along the way. It's incredible, isn't it? How even in our darkest moments, when we're grappling with the weight of grief, life has this way of teaching us lessons that are both beautiful and transformative. These lessons, learned in the crucible of loss, become part of our essence, shaping us into more compassionate, understanding, and resilient beings.

### The Impermanence of Life

One of the most striking lessons we learn is about the impermanence of life. It's a tough pill to swallow, realizing that everything and everyone we hold dear is only here for a limited time. But this awareness brings with it a certain clarity, a focus on what truly matters. It teaches us to cherish each moment, to live fully in the now, and not to take the people we love for granted. Like, have you ever noticed how, after losing someone, you hug your loved ones a little tighter, listen a bit more intently, and say "I love you" more often? That's this lesson at work.

### The Strength of the Human Spirit

Then there's the awe-inspiring resilience of the human spirit. If you had asked me before I went through loss whether I thought I could survive such heartache, I might have doubted my ability to endure. But here we are, continuing to live, love, and find joy despite the pain. This journey through loss shows us that we're capable of withstanding much more than we ever imagined. It's like discovering a well of strength within us that we didn't know existed until we had no choice but to draw from it.

## The Importance of Connection

Loss also teaches us about the importance of connection—how reaching out, sharing our grief, and supporting each other not only helps us heal but strengthens the bonds between us. It's in those moments of shared vulnerability that we find true connection, understanding, and compassion. It reminds us that no one is meant to navigate this life alone and that there's immense power in community and companionship. I've met people who, in their deepest grief, have forged friendships that are as solid as steel, all because they reached out in their moment of need.

## The Gift of Empathy

Through loss, we gain a profound sense of empathy. Having walked through the fire of grief, we're better able to understand and feel with others in their times of sorrow. It's as if our hearts expand, allowing us to hold space for others' pain alongside our own. This empathy moves us to act, to comfort, to be there for others in a way we might not have been before. It transforms us into a beacon of hope and support for those who are navigating their own storms.

### Finding Joy in Simplicity

Another beautiful lesson is finding joy in simplicity. In the wake of loss, the world's noise fades a bit, and we begin to find immense joy in the simplest of things—a shared meal, a walk in nature, a quiet moment alone with our thoughts. It's as if loss strips away the superficial, leaving us with a heightened appreciation for the beauty of the ordinary, the everyday. This shift in perspective is a gift, allowing us to live more fully, more gratefully.

### The Continuation of Love

Perhaps the most profound lesson of all is that love doesn't end with death. The love we have for those we've lost continues to thrive, to shape us, and to influence our lives in countless ways. It's a love that transcends physical presence, a bond that not even death can sever. This realization—that we carry our loved ones in our hearts, in our memories, and in the essence of who we are—offers comfort and a continuity that helps us navigate the journey ahead.

These lessons learned in the shadow of loss are not easy. They come at a great cost. But they're invaluable, shaping us into individuals who are more present, more compassionate, and more resilient. As we carry these lessons forward, they become our legacy, a testament to the enduring impact of the ones we've lost and the transformative power of grief and love.

So, as we reflect on these lessons, let's hold them close, allowing them to guide us, inspire us, and remind us of the beauty and fragility of life. In doing so, we honor those we've lost, not just in memory, but in the very way we choose to live our lives.

## 5.3 A New Chapter

Here we are, at a place that feels a bit like standing at the edge of a new dawn. It's that part of the journey where we talk about turning the page, about beginning A New Chapter. Now, I know, after everything we've been through—the loss, the grief, the moments of deep reflection—it might seem a bit daunting to think about what comes next. But trust me, this is where we start to see the light peeking through the clouds, where we begin to understand that our story continues, rich with the love and lessons from those we've lost.

### Embracing Change with Open Arms

One thing I've learned on this winding road is that life is all about change. Embracing this new chapter doesn't mean forgetting the past; it means carrying it with us as we step into the future. It's about holding tight to the memories and the love, letting them shape us as we embark on new adventures. Imagine you're setting sail on a vast ocean, the legacy of your loved ones like the wind in your sails, guiding you forward. It's a journey of discovery, of finding new passions, new joys, and perhaps even new ways to connect with the world around you.

## The Courage to Begin Again

Beginning again requires courage, no doubt about it. It's about giving yourself permission to seek happiness, to laugh, to love, without feeling guilty for moving forward. Remember, moving forward isn't moving on; it's simply allowing yourself to live fully, to embrace the complexity of holding grief in one hand and joy in the other. I've seen people start new hobbies, travel to places they've always dreamed of, or even change careers, all in the spirit of living a life that honors those they've lost by embracing the beauty of the present.

## Finding Joy in the Everyday

This new chapter is also about finding joy in the every day, in the small moments that fill our lives with color and light. It's about the morning coffee enjoyed in the quiet dawn, the laughter shared with friends, and the peace found in a good book or a walk in nature. These moments, seemingly simple, are where we find the strength to keep going, where we remember that life, despite its trials, is a beautiful gift.

## Building New Connections

As we navigate this new chapter, we also discover the power of building new connections. It's in these new friendships, new communities, that we find support, understanding, and companionship. It's not about replacing what was lost but about expanding our hearts to include new relationships that enrich our lives. These connections remind us that love is limitless and that our capacity to care, to connect, and to find kinship is one of our greatest strengths.

## The Legacy of Love Continues

Carrying the legacy of our loved ones into this new chapter is perhaps the most profound way we honor their memory. It's in the values we live by, the kindness we spread, and the love we share. Whether it's volunteering for a cause they were passionate about, continuing a tradition they started, or simply living each day with a bit more gratitude, we keep their spirit alive in the choices we make and the actions we take.

## A Renewed Sense of Purpose

This journey, with all its twists and turns, also has a way of revealing a renewed sense of purpose. It might come quietly, like the first light of dawn, or it might strike you in a moment of clarity. But when it arrives, it brings with it a sense of direction, a desire to make the most of the time we have, to leave our own mark on the world, inspired by the love and lessons of those we've lost.

## Welcoming the New Chapter

As we stand on the threshold of this new chapter, let's take a deep breath, let's embrace the uncertainty, the possibilities, the hope that lies ahead. Let's carry forward the love, the memories, the essence of those who have shaped us, letting them guide us as we write the next pages of our story.

This new chapter isn't about forgetting the past; it's about weaving it into the fabric of our future, creating a life that's rich with meaning, joy, and connection. It's about living fully, loving deeply, and moving forward with a heart full of gratitude for all that has been and all that is yet to come. So, here's to the new chapter, to the adventures it holds, and to the enduring power of love to light our way.

# Chapter 6

# Beyond Survival - Advocacy and

# Hope

Let's take a moment to appreciate how far we've come on this journey. From the heart-wrenching farewells to the profound lessons learned in the aftermath, it's been an emotional ride. Now, we're stepping into a realm that's all about transformation and transcendence—Chapter 6: Beyond Survival - Advocacy and Hope. It's here that we explore the powerful act of turning our pain into purpose.

### Turning Pain into Purpose

When the storm of grief begins to settle, a new dawn emerges for many of us. It's like we're standing at a crossroads, with the weight of our past and the possibility of our future stretching out before us. This is where pain meets purpose, where the deep ache of loss can morph into a force for change, advocacy, and hope.

### From Grief to Action

Imagine transforming the darkest moments of your life into a catalyst for change. It's about taking that swirling mass of grief, love, and memories and channeling it into something that not only honors your loved one but also makes a difference in the world. This is what advocacy is all about—fighting for a cause, championing a movement, or simply lending your voice to those who feel unheard.

Take, for example, the story of a father who lost his daughter to a rare form of cancer. Amid his deepest sorrow, he found a flicker of purpose in advocating for more research and better treatment options for the disease. He started a foundation in his daughter's name, turning his pain into a driving force behind a movement that now offers hope to countless others.

## The Ripple Effect of Advocacy

The beauty of turning pain into purpose through advocacy is the ripple effect it creates. It's like dropping a pebble into a pond—the initial impact might seem small, but the ripples spread far and wide, touching lives you may never even know about. Whether it's raising awareness, fundraising, or supporting others going through similar battles, your actions can inspire hope and bring about real change.

I've seen communities come together in incredible ways, rallying around causes started by individuals who, in their loss, found a mission. These movements not only serve as a living tribute to those they've lost but also as a beacon of hope for others. It's a testament to the power of the human spirit to find light in the darkness, to transform grief into action.

## Finding Your Path in Advocacy

Turning pain into purpose doesn't look the same for everyone. For some, it's about grand gestures and public movements. For others, it's quieter, more personal. Maybe it's volunteering your time, sharing your story to help others feel less alone, or simply living your life in a way that reflects the values and passions of the person you've lost.

The key is to find what resonates with you, what feels like a meaningful way to honor your loved one and make a difference. It might take time to discover what that looks like, and that's okay. The journey from pain to purpose is not a race; it's a path that unfolds in its own time, revealing opportunities for advocacy and hope in ways you might not expect.

## Hope as a Legacy

At the heart of advocacy lies hope—the belief that change is possible, that pain can give rise to purpose, and that our loved ones' legacies can fuel a brighter future. This hope is not just a comfort; it's a call to action. It's a promise to carry forward the love, the lessons, and the light of those we've lost, turning our shared experiences into a force for good.

As we navigate this chapter, let's embrace the possibility of turning our pain into purpose. Let's explore how advocacy can offer hope, not just to ourselves, but to the world. In doing so, we honor the memory of our loved ones, we connect with a community of like-minded souls, and we contribute to a legacy of change, compassion, and hope. It's a journey that reaffirms life's value and our capacity to rise, even from the deepest grief, with purpose and hope in our hearts.

## 6.2 Advances in Cancer Research

### A Dawn of Discovery

The landscape of cancer research is a testament to human ingenuity and perseverance. It's like watching the dawn break after a long, dark night. Each breakthrough, each advancement, brings with it a ray of hope, illuminating the possibilities of more tomorrows, of less pain, and of a future where cancer no longer holds the same power over us.

Imagine a world where the word "cancer" doesn't evoke the same fear it once did. This is the world that researchers, scientists, and medical professionals are tirelessly working towards. Through their dedication, we're witnessing incredible strides in understanding the mechanisms of cancer, leading to more targeted and effective treatments.

### The Power of Precision Medicine

One of the most exciting advancements is in the realm of precision medicine. It's like having a key crafted specifically for each lock, rather than using a one-size-fits-all approach. Precision medicine tailors treatment to the individual's genetic makeup, considering the specific mutations and characteristics of their cancer. This approach not only increases the effectiveness of the treatment but also minimizes the side effects, making the cancer journey less daunting for patients.

Take, for example, the development of targeted therapies and immunotherapies. These treatments have transformed the prognosis for certain types of cancer, turning what was once a death sentence into a manageable condition. It's nothing short of a revolution in cancer care, offering hope where there was once despair.

## The Role of Early Detection

Advancements in early detection are also changing the game. Through cutting-edge screening technologies and diagnostic tools, we're able to catch cancer at its earliest stages, significantly improving the chances of successful treatment. It's like spotting a storm on the horizon and having the means to prepare or even prevent it from hitting.

Research into biomarkers and imaging techniques is leading to earlier diagnoses, less invasive testing methods, and ultimately, better outcomes for patients. This progress not only saves lives but also spares countless individuals from the physical and emotional toll of undergoing aggressive treatments.

## The Promise of Personalized Vaccines

Imagine a future where we can not only treat cancer but prevent it through personalized vaccines. This isn't the stuff of science fiction but a reality that's becoming closer thanks to advances in cancer research. These vaccines, designed to train the immune system to recognize and fight cancer cells, are currently being tested and show immense promise. It's a groundbreaking approach that could redefine cancer prevention and treatment, offering a new layer of hope to individuals at risk.

## The Power of Collaboration

What makes these advances possible is not just the brilliance of individual researchers but the power of collaboration. Across the globe, scientists, institutions, and patients are coming together, sharing knowledge, resources, and experiences. This collective effort is accelerating the pace of discovery and bringing us closer to a future where cancer can be defeated.

The establishment of international consortia and the sharing of genetic data have opened new avenues for understanding cancer's complexities. It's a reminder that in the fight against cancer, we're stronger together, united by a common goal.

## The Fuel of Hope

As we explore the advances in cancer research, it's important to recognize the role of hope. Hope is not just a byproduct of scientific progress; it's the fuel that drives it. It's the hope for a cure, for a better quality of life, for more time with loved ones, that inspires researchers to push the boundaries of what's possible.

Hope is also what sustains patients and their families through the cancer journey. It's what encourages participation in clinical trials, support for research funding, and advocacy for better cancer care. It's a powerful force, capable of transforming pain into purpose, despair into determination.

## Looking Forward

As we look forward, the advancements in cancer research offer a beacon of hope, a promise of a future where cancer's shadow is less daunting. It's a testament to human resilience, to our capacity for innovation and compassion. While the journey is far from over, each step forward in research brings us closer to a world where cancer no longer steals our loved ones too soon.

As we wrap up this exploration of the advances in cancer research, let's hold onto hope, support the ongoing quest for discovery, and celebrate each victory along the way. Together, we're moving towards a future where cancer is no longer an end but a challenge that we can overcome, together.

## 6.3 A Community of Support

You know, if there's one silver lining to the cloud that is cancer, it's the incredible community of support that emerges from the struggle. It's like this vast network of warriors, survivors, caregivers, researchers, and supporters, all joined by a common cause: to face cancer head-on, not just to survive but to thrive, and to ensure no one has to walk this path alone.

### The Fabric of Support

Imagine this community as a giant quilt, each patch representing different forms of support—online forums, local support groups, nonprofit organizations, and cancer research advocates. Together, they create this warm, comforting blanket that wraps around anyone touched by cancer, offering solace, understanding, and hope.

### Online Havens

In today's digital age, support transcends physical boundaries. Online platforms have become havens where people from all corners of the globe connect. Here, you can share your story at 3 AM when sleep eludes you, or find a message of hope that brightens your darkest day. It's a space where advice, encouragement, and understanding flow freely, making the cancer journey feel less lonely.

### The Power of Local Groups

Local support groups, on the other hand, bring the comfort of physical presence. There's something about sitting in a circle with others who understand, sharing stories and tears, or even just nodding in silence, that heals the soul in ways words can't always express. These groups become families, bound not by blood but by shared experiences and the mutual desire to support each other through every high and low.

### Nonprofits and Advocacy

Then there are the nonprofits and advocacy groups, the backbone of the cancer support community. They're the ones pushing for more research, better treatments, and policies that support cancer patients and their families. They organize fundraising events, awareness campaigns, and offer resources that educate and empower. It's through their efforts that hope finds fertile ground to grow, promising a future where cancer no longer holds the power it once did.

### The Ripple Effect of Support

What's truly remarkable about this community of support is the ripple effect it creates. Every person who gives support, in turn, becomes a beacon of hope for others. It's a cycle of giving and receiving that strengthens not just individuals but the community as a whole. Like Emma, who, after losing her mother to cancer, started volunteering at a local cancer support organization. In helping others, she found a way to channel her grief into something positive, keeping her mother's spirit alive through acts of kindness.

## A Collective Strength

In this community, there's a collective strength that defies the odds. It's a force made up of countless individual stories of bravery, resilience, and love. Together, these stories weave a tapestry of hope that blankets the cancer journey, making it clear that no one has to face this battle alone.

## Hope Springs Eternal

And perhaps most importantly, this community is where hope springs eternal. Hope for a cure, hope for more birthdays, hope for a future where cancer is just a word in history books. It's in the research breakthroughs celebrated, the cancer anniversaries marked, and the simple, everyday victories that keep the flame of hope burning bright.

## Joining the Community

If you're walking the cancer journey, whether you're a patient, a survivor, a caregiver, or a loved one, know that this community is here for you. It's a place of refuge, a source of strength, and a wellspring of hope. And by joining this community, by sharing your own story, you not only find support but become a part of the support system for others.

As we talk about "A Community of Support," let's remember it's not just about fighting cancer; it's about building a world where compassion, understanding, and hope are the pillars that support us all. It's a reminder that together, we are stronger, and with each other's support, we can face anything—even cancer—with courage and hope.

# Conclusion

And just like that, we've journeyed together through the depths and peaks of a story that's both uniquely mine and, in so many ways, universally ours. From the first tremors of diagnosis, through the battles and the quiet moments of grace, to the final farewells and the delicate task of carrying forward the legacy of those we've loved and lost. Now, as we draw the curtains on this chapter of our collective journey, I want to sit with you for a moment, in the warm glow of a setting sun, and reflect on what this all means, on where we go from here.

This book, at its heart, is about love. It's about the kind of love that doesn't end with a last breath, the kind of love that fuels our fight against a relentless enemy, and the kind of love that keeps us standing when the world seems to crumble beneath our feet. It's about the love that continues to grow, even in our absence, shaping us, guiding us, and giving us the strength to face each new day.

But it's also about resilience—the incredible capacity of the human spirit to endure pain, to adapt to unimaginable loss, and to find a way to blossom in the aftermath. We've seen that resilience isn't just about withstanding the storm; it's about learning to dance in the rain, to find beauty in the brokenness, and to forge meaning from the ashes of our grief.

As we close this chapter, I want to remind you that the end of this book is not the end of the story. It's merely a new beginning, a stepping stone to a future where our pain becomes our purpose, where our losses illuminate our paths, and where the love we've shared continues to inspire and guide us.

I invite you to look at your own journey through the lens of hope. Yes, cancer is a formidable foe, and yes, the path is often fraught with uncertainty and pain. But it's also lined with moments of incredible beauty, deep connections, and opportunities for growth and transformation. Our stories are testaments to the power of hope, to the belief that, even in the darkest of times, there's a light that can guide us home.

Let's carry forward the lessons we've learned, not as burdens, but as beacons. Let's share our stories, not as tales of sorrow, but as sagas of survival, resilience, and hope. And let's continue to support one another, not because we've walked the same path, but because we understand the journey's weight and the strength found in unity.

The community of support we've built, the advances in cancer research we've witnessed, and the advocacy we've championed are all proof that, together, we are stronger than cancer. They are reminders that, while we may not have chosen this path, we have the power to shape where it leads, to make a difference in the lives of those who walk it with us, and to contribute to a future where cancer no longer holds the power to dictate our stories.

As we look to the horizon, let's do so with hearts full of love, spirits brimming with resilience, and minds open to the endless possibilities that lie ahead. Let's live our lives in a way that honors those we've lost, cherishing their memories, carrying forward their legacies, and embodying the lessons they've taught us.

This journey, with all its pain, beauty, and complexity, is a reminder of what it means to be human. It's a call to embrace life in all its fragility, to love deeply, to face each challenge with courage, and to never lose sight of hope.

So, as we part ways, remember that you are not alone. You are part of a vast, vibrant community bound by shared experiences, common struggles, and collective hope. Together, we've weathered the storm, navigated the aftermath, and emerged with a renewed sense of purpose and possibility.

Thank you for walking this path with me, for sharing in the tears, the laughter, and the love. As you turn the pages of your own story, may you do so with the knowledge that, even in the darkest nights, the dawn is always within reach. Here's to the journey ahead, to the stories yet to be written, and to the enduring power of love and hope that guides us, always.

With all my heart, **Rae Make**r.